Preface

The standard of World Federation of Acupuncture – Moxibustion Societies, which is put forward by World Federation of Acupuncture – Moxibustion Societies in accordance with the general requirements of sterile acupuncture needles for single use (refers to Filiform Needles), of clinical practice, and of medical devices.

The adjusted standard is based on WFAS standard 001: 2011 and the recommendations from Standard committee members. The main change is to delete the contents of the un – sterilized acupuncture needles (reusable acupuncture needles that a practitioner must sterilize before each use).

Details of the modifications are as follows:

1. Deleting the relevant contents of the un – sterilized acupuncture needles in the first paragraph in the *"Introduction"*.

2. Revising *"1 Scope"*, deleted the relevant contents of the un – sterilized acupuncture needles. The standard applies to the sterile acupuncture needles for single use (refers to Filiform Needles).

3. Deleting the original clause 4. 2: *"The varieties of acupuncture needles include un – sterilized acupuncture needles (reusable acupuncture needles that a practitioner must sterilize before each use) and sterile acupuncture needles (acupuncture needles for single use)."*

4. Revising TABLE 5 *"Hardness of the Needle Body"*, TABLE 7 *"Appearance Quality and Ra Value"* and TABLE 8 *"Pulling Force"*, deleted the relevant contents of the un – sterilized acupuncture needles.

5. Revising the original clause 8. 1: *"Primary package: the information of Sterile Acupuncture Needle for single use should be on the label of the sterile primary package."*

6. Revising the original clause 8. 2: *"Secondary package: the labels should be on the secondary package of Sterile Acupuncture Needles for single use."*

7. Serial numbers of the chapters were re – adjusted.

Annex A, Annex B and Annex C of this standard are normative.

Annex D of this standard is informative.

The drafting Units: Suzhou Medical Appliance Factory, China.

Main drafters: Cao Yang, Xu Aimin, Jiang Xinsui.

Members of the International working group: James Flowers (Australia), Wu Binjiang (Canada), Cao Yang (China), Huang Longxiang (China), Liu Baoyan (China), Tan Yuansheng (China), Denis Colin (France), Francois Dumont (France), Andreas Rinnoessel (Germany), Sergio Bangrazi (Italy), Cho Geun Sik (Korea), Liao Chunhua (Malaysia), Liu Yun (USA).

International observers: Naoto Ishizaki (Japan).

U0346128

Introduction

The Standard applies to Sterile Acupuncture Needles for single use (refers to Filiform Needles) used by professional acupuncturists. The sterile acupuncture needles for single are sterilized before leaving the factory in order to guarantee that the product is germ – free, the healthcare professional can open the sealed package and use the needle immediately.

In order to encourage innovation, the standard will no longer enforce the combination of the needle diameter and length. However, considering the clinical usage requirements, the standard provides the specifications for the needle diameter and length.

The sharpness and puncture performance of the needle tip are of a very important clinical significance. Annex A states the guidelines and the evaluation methods for the strength and the sharpness of the needle tip, while Annex B provides two qualitative and quantitative evaluation methods to determine the tip's puncture performance.

The qualitative methods to evaluate the tip's puncture performance are described in Annex B. The methods are simple, direct and practical. It makes them especially suitable for the routine inspection and for the cross-comparison of the acupuncture needles clinical applications. They also play a very important role in the enhancement of the quality of the acupuncture needle tip. The methods to evaluate the puncture performance of the needle tip can be used to further evaluate the puncture and puncture performance of the acupuncture needle. Currently, the more appropriate method is to use the needle tip to pierce through polyurethane material; however, this method has not yet been implemented internationally. Considering the consistency of standards in the future, this standard provides the methods to evaluate the puncture performance of the needle tip and ranks Clause 5.4.2 as a recommendatory one. The standard does not provide the sharpness index of the piercing through polyurethane material by the needle tip. This index will be added to the standard when it becomes appropriate. To improve product quality, all inspection reports should include the inspection information as well as the results of the performance evaluation.

Since every manufacturer's design, production, and sterilization methods are different, no regulations exist for the materials of the acupuncture needle handle. Still, the needle body and the needle handle of acupuncture needle should have good biocompatibility. The guidance for the biological evaluation of the medical devices given in ISO 10993 – 1 should be applied. It is highly advised that the manufacturer adheres to the guidelines when evaluating their products in order to enhance their quality. The evaluation should include the effect of the sterilization process on the acupuncture needle.

At the same time, in order to ensure product safety and efficacy, the manufacturer should perform risk analysis and enforce risk management in addition to adhering to the requirements of local rules and regulations, the relevant background data of the medical devices and clinical practice throughout the entire duration of the product's life cycle. ISO 14971 has provided manufacturers a framework for the effective management of hazards associated with the use of medical devices.

In some countries, the requirements proposed here are subject to legal sanctions. Such rules and regulations should take precedence over the standards set forth in this document.

Introduction

1 Scope

The standard specifies the requirements for the classification, criteria, test methods, inspection rules, packaging, labelling, instructions for use, transport, storage for the sterile acupuncture needles for single use.

The standard applies to the sterile acupuncture needles for single use (refers to Filiform Needles).

2 Normative References

The following references are indispensable for the proper application of the corresponding standards. For dated references, only the edition cited applies. For undated references, the latest edition of the referenced document (including any amendments) applies.

ISO/TS 15510: 2007 Stainless steels – Chemical composition

ISO 10993 – 1: 2009 Biological evaluation of medical devices – Part 1: Evaluation and experiment in the process of risk management

ISO 6507 – 1: 2005 Metallic materials – Vickers hardness test – Part 1: Test method

ISO 11737 – 2: 2007 Sterilization of medical devices – Microbiological methods – Part 2: Tests of sterility performed in the validation of a sterilization process

ISO 15223 – 1 Medical devices – Symbols to be used with medical device labels, labelling and information to be supplied – Part 1: General requirements

3 Terms and Definitions

Forthe purposes of this document, the following terms and definitions apply.

3. 1 Body of the Needle

The part of the acupuncture needle that is inserted into the body (Figure 1).

3. 2 Handle of the Needle

The part of the acupuncture needle that is not inserted into the body (Figure 1).

3. 3 Tip of the Needle

The sharp apex at the end of the acupuncture needle body is inserted into the body (Figure 1).

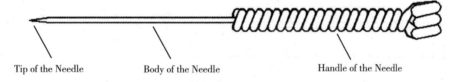

Tip of the Needle   Body of the Needle   Handle of the Needle

Figure 1 Typical Structure of Acupuncture Needle

3. 4 Root of the Needle

The part of the acupuncture needle that connects the needle body to the needle handle (Figure 1).

3. 5 Tail of the Needle

The end part of the needle handles at the opposite side of the needle apex (Figure 1).

3. 6 Sterile Acupuncture Needles

The acupuncture needles that have been sterilized.

3. 7 Un – sterilized Acupuncture Needles

The acupuncture needles that have not been sterilized.

3. 8 Guide Tube

An assistant tool inthe shape of slender, long tube into which the needle is put and used for easy inserting.

Note: In order to facilitate the use, guide tube should be made of transparent materials.

3.9 Hardness of Needle Body

The body of acupuncture needle has a characteristic of resisting permanent deformation.

3.10 Primary Package

The material that first envelops the product and holds it.

Note: This usually is the smallest unit package of use and is the package which is in direct contact with a piece or several pieces of acupuncture needles.

3.11 Secondary Package

The package of several primary packages for distribution and keeping.

4 Classification

4.1 The configuration of the acupuncture needle and the name of each of its parts are shown in Figure 1.

4.2 The acupuncture needle includes two types, one with guide tube and another without guide tube. The acupuncture needle with guide tube is shown in Figure 2.

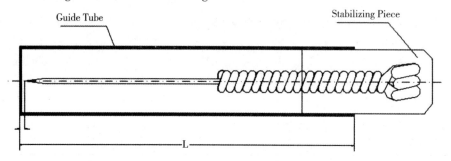

Figure 2　Sterile Acupuncture Needle (with Guide Tube)

Note: No uniform requirement is provided for the fixing method of needle tube as shown in Figure 2.

4.3 The types of needle handles are the ring handle, the plain handle, the flower handle, the metal tube handle, and the plastic handle. The types of acupuncture needles are shown in Figure 3 below.

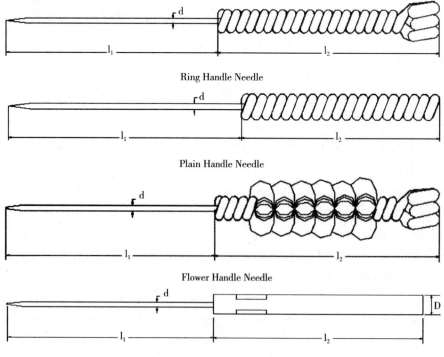

Ring Handle Needle

Plain Handle Needle

Flower Handle Needle

Metal Tube Handle Needle

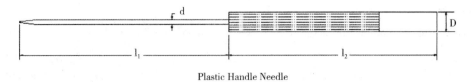

Plastic Handle Needle

d: diameter of needle body

D: diameter of needle handle

l_1: length of needle body

l_2: length of needle handle

Figure3　The Types of Acupuncture Needles

Note: The types of needles in the above figure show certain kinds of typical structures. There are no uniform regulations regarding the method of using guide tubes to stabilize the needle.

4.4　The specifications of the acupuncture needle are marked as: needle diameter × needle length.

Example: φ0.30mm × 40mm

4.5　The basic dimensions and tolerance of acupuncture needles should comply with Tables 1 ~ 4.

4.5.1　The needle diameter should comply with Table 1.

Table 1　Basic Measurement of Needle Diameter (mm)

Needle Diameter of Standard Range (d)	Allowable Difference
$0.12 \leqslant d < 0.25$	±0.008
$0.25 \leqslant d \leqslant 0.45$	±0.015
$0.45 < d \leqslant 0.80$	±0.020

4.5.2　The needle length should comply with Table 2.

Table 2　Basic Measurement of Needle Length (mm)

Needle Length of Standard Range (l_1)	Allowable Difference
$5 < l_1 \leqslant 25$	±0.50
$25 < l_1 \leqslant 75$	±1.00
$75 < l_1 \leqslant 150$	±1.50
$100 < l_1 \leqslant 200$	±2.00

4.5.3　The length of the needle handle should be no less than 13mm.

4.5.4　The specifications of the coiling handle wire should comply with Table 3. The diameter of the plastic handle and the metal tube handle should comply with Table 4.

Table 3　Diameter of the Coiling Handle Wire (mm)

Needle Diameter of Standard Range (d)	Diameter of Coiling Handle Wire
$0.12 \leqslant d < 0.20$	0.30
$0.20 \leqslant d < 0.30$	0.35
$0.30 \leqslant d < 0.40$	0.40
$0.40 \leqslant d < 0.50$	0.45

Table 4　Diameter of the Plastic Handle and the Metal Tube Handle (mm)

Type of Needle Handle	Handle Diameter (d)
Metal Tube Handle, Plastic Handle, etc.	0.80 ~ 2.50

5　Requirements

5. 1　The basic dimensions of the acupuncture needle should comply with the specifications listed in Clause 4. 5.

5. 2　There is no uniform regulation regarding the material of the needle handle and body. It should be of good biocompatibility. Currently, the popularly used needle body material is made of X5CrNi18 – 9, X7CrNi18 – 9 Austenite Stainless Steel etc are given in ISO/TS 15510: 2007.

Note: When the material of the acupuncture needle body has been altered, there will be an additional coating (such as Lubricant) on the surface of the needle body or there will be evidence indicating that it can cause harmful side effects to the human body. In such circumstances, in accordance with ISO 10993 – 1: 2009 for guidance on biocompatibility, it is necessary to perform biological evaluation of the material and the final product. The basic evaluation and testing are:

　　　a. Cytotoxicity;

　　　b. Sensitization;

　　　c. Intracutaneous Reactivity;

　　　d. Ethylene oxide sterilization residuals (if using EO. to sterilize).

5. 3　The hardness of the needle body should comply with the specifications in Table 5.

Table 5　Hardness of the Needle Body

Needle Diameter of Standard Range (d, mm)	Hardness ($HV_{0.2kg}$)
$0.12 \leqslant d < 0.25$	$\geqslant 480, \leqslant 650$
$0.25 \leqslant d \leqslant 0.30$	$\geqslant 460, \leqslant 650$
$0.30 < d \leqslant 0.45$	$\geqslant 450, \leqslant 650$
$0.45 < d \leqslant 0.80$	$\geqslant 420, \leqslant 530$

5. 4　The intensity and puncture performance of the needle tip.

5. 4. 1　The tip of the acupuncture needle should be round and without defects, and it should have good strength. The needle tip should not have any hooks or bends after a set amount of pressure has been applied. The puncture force should not exceed the values set forth in Table 6.

Table 6　Pressure and Puncture Force

Needle Diameter of Standard Range (d, mm)	Pressure (N)	Puncture Force (N)
$0.12 \leqslant d < 0.25$	0.4	0.7
$0.25 \leqslant d \leqslant 0.30$	0.5	0.8
$0.30 < d \leqslant 0.45$	0.6	0.9
$0.45 < d \leqslant 0.80$	0.7	1.0

5. 4. 2　The tip of the acupuncture needle should be round and without defects, and it should have good puncture performance.

5. 5　The acupuncture needle should be of sufficient toughness, and it should not exhibit any cracks, breaks or separation of layers after the winding test.

5. 6　The needle surface should be smooth, clean and free of any defect or foreign matter produced during the metal processing course and its appearance quality and coarseness parameter (Ra value) should comply with Table 7.

Table 7   Appearance Quality and Ra Value

Appearance Quality	Should not have any obvious defects such as scars, bends, or fine scratches
Ra value	$\leq 0.63\,\mu m$

5.7   The point at which the needle handle and body connects should be firm and sturdy, and both axial displacements should be no more than 3 mm during the pulling test by the force values shown in Table 8.

Table 8   Pulling Force

Needle Diameter of Standard Range (d, mm)	Pulling Force (N)
$0.12 \leq d \leq 0.18$	7
$0.18 < d \leq 0.25$	9
$0.25 < d \leq 0.30$	14
$0.30 < d \leq 0.45$	19
$0.45 < d \leq 0.80$	24

5.8   If the needle handle is made with winding coils, the spiral loop should be arranged symmetrically without obvious gaps.

5.9   The needle handle should not have any protuberances.

5.10   The acupuncture needle should be straight and without obvious bends or curves.

5.11   The color and luster of the surface of the needle handle should be even. If the handle is made with plating, it should not exhibit layering or shedding.

5.12   No visible microsphere is formed on the surface of needle when observed with normal or corrected visual acuity if lubricant is applied to the needle body.

5.13   The needle body should have good corrosion resistance.

5.14   Sterile Acupuncture Needles should be sterilized through a confirmed sterilization procedure in order to assure that the products are sterile.

Note: For appropriate sterilization methods, see Annex D. The Requirements for validation and routine control of a sterilization process for medical devices are provided in ISO 11135 – 1: 2007, ISO 11137 – 1: 2006 and ISO 17665 – 1: 2006 should apply.

6   Test Methods

6.1   Appearance

Inspect with the naked eye or corrected visual acuity or with a 10 times magnifier.

6.2   Surface Coarseness

Inspect with the naked eye or corrected visual acuity or with a 10 times magnifier, compare with the surface coarseness sample.

6.3   Measurement

Measure using general and specialized measuring tools.

6.4   Function

6.4.1   Hardness Test

Assess the hardness test according to the requirements given in ISO 6507 – 1: 2005, which should comply with Clause 5.3.

6.4.2   Test for Needle Tip Strength, Sharpness and Puncture Performance

Perform the tests according to the requirements noted in Annex A and B, which should comply with clauses 5.4.1 and 5.4.2, respectively.

6.4.3 Test for Resilience of the Needle Body.

The needle body should be encircled by a tight coil along the direction of a helical line in the central axis with the diameter of 3 times that of the needle body. The needle body should be wound by two circles if the needle body length is ≤15mm and by five circles if the needle body length is any of the other specifications, which should comply with Clause 5.5.

6.4.4 Test for the Firmness of the Connecting between the Needle Body and the Handle

Firstly, measure the length of the needle body in advance, then affix the needle body in the clamp. Perform the non – impactive pulling test along the axis of the needle body on the surface of the needle handle according to Clause 5.7. Afterwards, the needle length should be measured again according to Clause 5.7.

6.4.5 Test for Protuberances on the Needle Handle

When touching the needle handle with the hands, there should be no detectable protuberances according to Clause 5.9.

6.4.6 Test for the Corrosive Nature of the Needle Body

Test for the corrosive nature according to the requirements noted in Annex C, which should comply with Clause 5.13.

6.4.7 Test of Sterility

Tests of sterility performed in the validation of a sterilization process according to the requirements given in ISO 11737 – 2: 2007, Sterile Acupuncture needles should comply with Clause 5.14.

7 Packaging

7.1 Primary package of sterile acupuncture needles should be well sealed; the package should not contain any foreign objects visible to the naked eye. The material and design of the package should be ensured and should not cause any damage to the product contained within:

a. When stored in dry, clean, and sufficiently ventilated conditions, the products should be guaranteed to be sterile when used before the expiration date.

b. The packaged product should be exposed to minimal contamination risk when being removed from the package.

c. During normal transference, transport, and storage, the packaged product should be fully protected.

d. Once the package has been opened, it can no longer be easily resealed, and thus it should have noticeable traces of tear when opened.

Note: The Requirements for materials, sterile barrier systems and packaging systems for terminally sterilized medical devices are provided by ISO 11607 and EN 868. The content of the standard should be considered by the manufacturer during the evaluation and design of the packaging of sterile acupuncture needles.

7.2 Primary Package should guarantee that the acupuncture needles will not rust before the expiration date.

7.3 Secondary Package is the smallest package unit for inspection and distribution.

7.4 Out package should be secure enough to ensure that the products will remain undamaged during normal transport and storage and that the labels or marking should remain clear and legible for many years.

8 Labelling

8.1 Primary Package

The following information should be on the label of both the primary package at least:

a. Manufacturer's name and (or) trademark;

b. Name of product;

c. Specifications;

d. Quantity (if applicable) ;

e. Date of manufacture and (or) batch number;

f. Method of sterilization, the word "sterile" and (or) symbol;

g. The words "For single use" or "Do not reuse" and (or) symbol;

h. Expiration date.

8.2   Secondary Package

The same type and specifications for primary package of acupuncture needles should be shown on the secondary package, along with the following information at least:

a. Manufacturer's name, address and trademark;

b. Name of product;

c. Type, specifications and quantity;

d. Date of manufacture and (or) batch number;

e. Certificate number according to the requirements of the regulations;

f. Method of sterilization, the word "Sterile" and (or) symbol;

g. The words "For single use" or "Do not reuse" and (or) symbol;

h. Expiration date;

i. If appropriate, that the name or composition of additive (such as Lubricant) are coated on the surface of needle body.

j. Warning: Those who are allergic tothe material of needle body should make use with caution or following the instruction of an acupuncture physician; Electrical stimulation is possible to produce corrosion to needles; use is prohibited if package is broken; destroy (by melting / burning) after use.

Before use, check to see that warnings are onthe secondary package, unless such warnings are already primary package.

8.3   The labels, symbols, and information on the packaging should comply with ISO 15223 − 1.

8.4   Revisions of the instructions for use should comply with Medical Devices Regulatory.

9   Storage and Transport

9.1   The transport requirements should comply with the order contract.

9.2   After packaging, the acupuncture needles should be stored in a clean, well − ventilated, non − contaminated environment with a relative humidity level of no more than 80%. The needles should have sufficient protection from damage.

Annex A

(Normative)

Test Methods for the Strength and Sharpness of the Acupuncture Needle Tip

A. 1 Definitions

The strength of the acupuncture needle tip: refers to the needle's ability to resist breakage when thrust vertically on the steel block.

The sharpness of the acupuncture needle tip: refers to the force required by the needle tip to vertically pierce the aluminum foil.

A. 2 Apparatus for Measuring the Strength and Sharpness of the Acupuncture Needle Tip

The apparatus (Figure A1) should comply with the following requirements and should be manufactured according to the design and documents approved by the regulated procedure.

A. 2. 1 The unit of the sharpness of the needle tip's puncture force is shown as "N".

A. 2. 2 The full load, minimum value and speed of the apparatus should comply with Table A1.

Table A1   The Full Load, Minimum Value and Speed of the Apparatus

Items	Designation
Full Load	1. 2N
Minimum Value	0. 01N
Speed	≤0. 1mm/s

A. 2. 3 The apparatus's erroneous differences in value should be no more than 0. 01N.

A. 2. 4 The apparatus should have an auto – correction capability and an antishock device. The needle clamp should be stable during use.

A. 2. 5 The transmission of the apparatus should be sensitive and reliable. The pointer should stop automatically when it pierces through the aluminum foil and meets the electrode.

A. 2. 6 The starting inductive quantity of the apparatus should be no more than 0. 02N.

A. 3 The Steel Block of the Strength of the Sample Acupuncture Needle Tip

The steel block surface of the strength of the sample acupuncture needle tip should be smooth and without rust.

A. 4 The Aluminum Foil of the Measuring Apparatus Used to Test the Sharpness of the Acupuncture Needle Tip

A. 4. 1 The aluminum foil surface should be clean and smooth and without overlaps, severe wrinkles, mildew stains, or sand holes.

A. 4. 2 The aluminum foil is a pliable material. The thickness should be 0. 05mm with deviations of ±0. 002mm and purity of no less than 99. 5%.

A. 4. 3 The strength of the pull resistance of the aluminum foil should be no less than 3 kg/mm^2, and the tensility rate should be no less than 3%.

A. 5 Test Methods

A. 5. 1 Testing the strength of the needle tip: After the test sample is affixed to the apparatus (with 5mm of the acupuncture needle tip exposed), the needle tip is thrust vertically onto the steel block. According to the rule in A. 2. 2, increase force, speed and load until they reach the numerical values of the standard set by 5. 4. 1, removing the load after 5 seconds. Then, observe the sample under a 5 times magnifying glass. The needle tip should not have any bends or hooks. In addition, when the needle tip is dragged along the surface of sterilized cotton, it should not pull any fibers.

A. 5. 2 After the strength test, keep the sample acupuncture needle clamped in the test apparatus and allow the needle to gradually increase its force exerted on the aluminum foil (by way of the transmission); the swaying rod will react accordingly. When the force acting on the acupuncture needle exceeds the resistance of the aluminum foil, the needle tip will pierce through the aluminum foil and come into contact with the electrode. The apparatus will automatically stop increasing the force. At this time, the value indicated by the pointer on the swaying rod is the piercing force of the needle tip.

A. 5. 3 Press the on – off button of the function controls to allow the swaying rod and pointer to return to their original positions.

A. 5. 4 Move the aluminum foil in the clamp to allow the diameter of each pierced hole to exceed three times that of the test sample.

A. 5. 5 Repeat the above steps, A. 5. 2, A. 5. 3 and A. 5. 4; measure 3 times to obtain the average values.

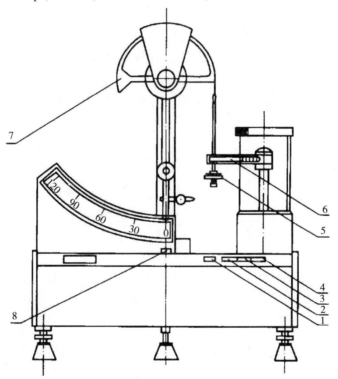

1: power button (on and off)

2, 3, 4: function control button (on and off)

5: aluminum foil clamping apparatus

6: needle clamping apparatus

7: adjustment rod

8: (carpenter's) level

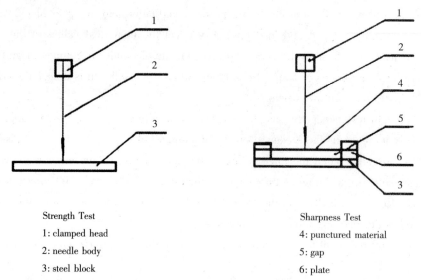

Strength Test

1: clamped head

2: needle body

3: steel block

Sharpness Test

4: punctured material

5: gap

6: plate

Figure A1   The Principles of the Method of Testing for the Sharpness and Strength of the Needle Tip

Annex B

(Normative)

Test Methods for the Puncture Performance of the Acupuncture Needle Tip

B. 1   Method 1: Test Method of the Qualitative

Coverthe mouth of a cup (diameter of 100mm) with the membrane of surgical rubber gloves (in accordance with ISO 10282: 2002) and tighten it properly with a rubber band. Puncture the membrane perpendicularly with the acupuncture needle. During the piercing, if the dent of the membrane is small and there is little resistance, this indicates that the needle tip is sharp. Otherwise, the needle tip is blunt.

Note: This method can be qualitatively evaluated depending on the needle's puncture performance. This method is suitable for the cross – comparison of the purchaser and the quality control of production.

B. 2   Method 2: Test Method of the Quantitative

B. 2. 1   The Testing Apparatus for Evaluating Puncture Force

Figure B1 is a sketch map produced bythe typical apparatus for measuring and recording puncture force. Other apparatuses of similar performance and precision can also be used. The apparatus should provide the following:

a. Speed V = (50 ~ 250) mm/min, the average drive precision ≤ established drive speed ±5%.

b. Average precision of the (0 ~ 50) sensor is ±5% of full range.

c. Puncture diameter of polymerized film after clamping is 10mm.

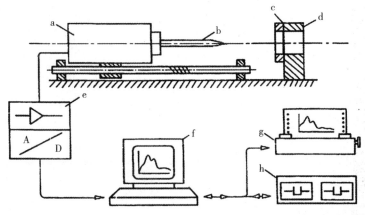

Figure B1   Sketch Map Produced by the Typical Testing Apparatus for Puncture Performance Evaluation

B. 2. 2   The Polymerized Film Materials

The polymerized wax suitable for the piercing test is elastic with a thickness of 0. 35 ±0. 05mm. The Shore Hardness of the polyurethane film is 85 ±10HA.

B. 2. 3   The Steps for Evaluating Puncture Force

B. 2. 3. 1   The polymerized film is placed in 22 °C ± 2 °C for 24 hours and tested in the same temperature.

B. 2. 3. 2   One part of the polymerized film C of sequent length is clamped vertically on the apparatus DK. The polymerized film should not be tense. If the polymerized film has a refined processing surface, this surface should face the needle tip.

B. 2. 3. 3   The handle of the test acupuncture needle is installed on the fixed apparatus and the needle body

15

is placed perpendicularly to the surface of the polymerized film. The needle tip points to the center of the round puncture area.

B. 2. 3. 4   The movement speed is 100mm/min.

B. 2. 3. 5   Turn on the testing apparatus.

B. 2. 3. 6   Pierce the polymerized film and record the graph of force versus corresponding displacement.

B. 2. 3. 7   Measure the corresponding peak values (F_0, F_1 and F_2).

B. 2. 3. 8   Unused and non – punctured areas should be selected during every piercing of the polymerized film.

B. 2. 4   Recording the Peak Values of the Coordinate Figures

The various force values can be identified by observing the typical peak values during the puncturing of the polymerized film by the needle.

F_0: The peak force of the needle tip piercing through the polymerized film.

F_1: The peak force of the slanted surface of the needle tip cutting through the polymerized film.

F_2: The frictional peak force of the length of the needle body piercing through the polymerized film.

B. 3   The Results Indicate

Compare with the same types of needles (of known quality and performance) to evaluate the coordinate graph of differences in force and position.

B. 4 and B. 5 provide the typical coordinate figures as well as the method for reporting the results of the test.

B. 4   Diagram of the Typical Features of the Needle Piercing Through the Film

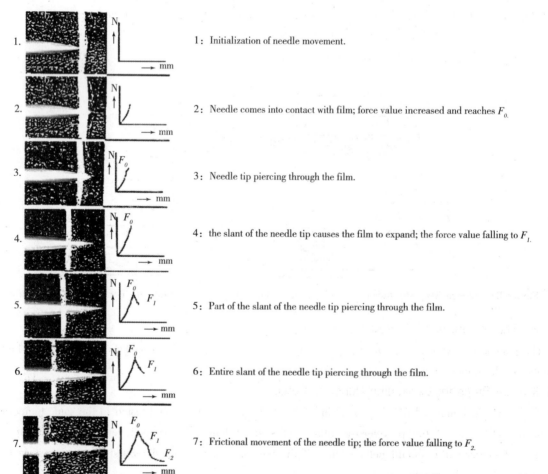

1: Initialization of needle movement.

2: Needle comes into contact with film; force value increased and reaches F_0.

3: Needle tip piercing through the film.

4: the slant of the needle tip causes the film to expand; the force value falling to F_1.

5: Part of the slant of the needle tip piercing through the film.

6: Entire slant of the needle tip piercing through the film.

7: Frictional movement of the needle tip; the force value falling to F_2.

B. 5 Diagram of the Needle's Typical Puncture Force (F_0、 F_1、 F_2)

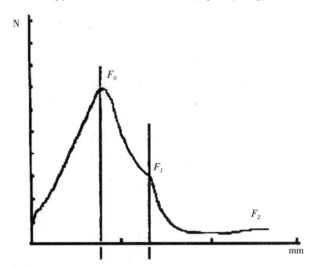

Annex C

(Normative)

Test Method for Corrosion Resistance——Testing with Citric Acid Solution

C. 1   Test Instruments

Glass beaker.

C. 2   Reagent

Citric acid (pure).

C. 3   Preparation

C. 3. 1   Test Water

The test water is the grade 3 water stipulated in ISO 3696.

C. 3. 2   Citric Acid Solution Compound

The citric acid solution is mixed with 100g/L (10%) of the grade 3 water.

C. 3. 3   Preparation

Any grease or dirt should be wiped off of the Austenitic stainless steel of the needle body or manufactured needle body. After wiping, the test articles can be soaked in acetone or other organic solutions for further degreasing. Then, the articles should be washed and rinsed with the grade 3 water and set aside in preparation for later use.

C. 4   Test Procedure

C. 4. 1   Soak test articles in the citric acid solution and keep them in a room – temperature environment for five hours.

C. 4. 2   Remove the articles from the solution and wash them with the grade 3 water.

C. 4. 3   Place the articles in the glass beaker with the grade 3 water and boil for 30 minutes.

C. 4. 4   Allow the articles to cool off in the test water and keep them in a room – temperature setting for 48 hours.

C. 4. 5   Remove the articles from the test water and place them in an airy environment for natural evaporation to dry or blow – dry them with hot air.

C. 5   Test Evaluation

Traces of corrosion onthe article's surface should be examined by the naked eye or with a 10 times magnifier. The degree of corrosion should be of rustless phenomena.

Annex D

(Informative)

References

[1] ISO 780: 1997, Packaging – Pictorial marking for handling of goods

[2] ISO 2859 – 1: 1999, Sampling procedures for inspection by attributes – Part 1: Sampling schemes indexed by acceptance quality limit (AQL) for lot – by – lot inspection

[3] ISO 3696: 1987, Water for analytical laboratory use – Specification and test methods

[4] ISO 6507 – 1: 2005, Metallic materials – Vickers hardness test – Part 1: Test method

[5] ISO 6507 – 2: 2005, Metallic materials – Vickers hardness test – Part 2: Verification and calibration of testing machines

[6] ISO 6507 – 3: 2005, Metallic materials – Vickers hardness test – Part 3: Calibration of reference blocks

[7] ISO 6507 – 4: 2005, Metallic materials – Vickers hardness test – Part 4: Tables of hardness values

[8] ISO 7864: 1993, Sterile hypodermic needles for single use

[9] ISO 7000: 1989, Graphical symbols for use one equipment – Index and synopsis

[10] ISO 10282: 2002, Single – use sterile rubber surgical glovers – Specification

[11] ISO 10993 – 1: 2009, Biological evaluation of medical devices – Part 1 Evaluation and testing within a risk management process

[12] ISO 10993 – 5: 2009, Biological evaluation of medical devices – Part 5: Tests for in vitro cytotoxicity

[13] ISO 10993 – 7: 2008, Biological evaluation of medical devices – Part 7: Ethylene oxide sterilization residuals

[14] ISO 10993 – 10: 2010, Biological evaluation of medical devices – Part 10: Tests for irritation and skin sensitization

[15] ISO 10993 – 11: 2006, Biological evaluation of medical devices – Part 11: Tests for systemic toxicity

[16] ISO 11135 – 1: 2007, Sterilization of health care products – Ethylene oxide – Part 1: Requirements for development, validation and routine control of a sterilization process for medical devices

[17] ISO 11137 – 1: 2006, Sterilization of health care products – Radiation – Part 1: Requirements for development, validation and routine control of a sterilization process for medical devices

[18] ISO 11137 – 2: 2006, Sterilization of health care products – Radiation – Part 2: Establishing the sterilization dose

[19] ISO 11138 – 1: 2006, Sterilization of health care products – Biological indicators – Part 1: General requirements

[20] ISO 11138 – 2: 2006, Sterilization of health care products – Biological indicators – Part 2: Biological indicators for ethylene oxide sterilization processes

[21] ISO 11607 – 1: 2006, Packaging for terminally sterilized medical devices – Part 1: Requirements for materials, sterile barrier systems and packaging systems

[22] ISO 11607 – 2: 2006, Packaging for terminally sterilized medical devices – Part 2: Validation requirements for forming, sealing and assembly processes

[23] ISO 11737 – 1: 2006, Sterilization of medical devices – Microbiological methods – Part 1: Determination of a population of microorganisms on products

WFAS STANDARD 001 : 2013

[24] ISO 11737 – 2 – 2007, Sterilization of medical devices – Microbiological methods – Part 2: Tests of sterility performed in the validation of a sterilization process

[25] ISO 13485: 2003, Medical devices – Quality management systems – Requirements for regulatory purposes

[26] ISO 14971: 2007, Medical Devices – Application of risk management to medical devices

[27] ISO 15223 – 1: 2007, Medical devices – Symbols to be used with medical device labels, labelling and information to be supplied – Part 1: General requirements

[28] ISO 15223 – 2: 2010, Medical devices – Symbols to be used with medical device labels, labelling, and information to be supplied – Part 2: Symbol development, selection and validation

[29] ISO/TS 15510: 2007, Stainless steels – Chemical composition

[30] ISO 17665 – 1: 2006, Sterilization of health care products – Moist heat – Part 1: Requirements for the development, validation and routine control of a sterilization process for medical devices

[31] EN 980: 2008, Graphical Symbols for Use in the Labelling of Medical Devices

[32] EN 1041: 2008, Information Supplied by the Manufacturer with Medical Devices

[33] EN 10088 – 1: 2005, Stainless steels

[34] GB/T 1031 – 1995, Surface roughness parameters andtheir values

[35] GB 2024 – 1994, Acupuncture needles

[36] GB/DRT 2024 – 2010, Acupuncture needles (Draft standard)

[37] GB 15811 – 2001, Sterile hypodermic needles for single use

[38] GB 15980 – 1995, Hygienic standard of disinfection for single use medical products

[39] YY 0043 – 2005, Medical suture needle

[40] YY 0033 – 2000, Good manufacture practice for sterile medical devices

[41] YY/T 0149 – 2006, Stainless steel medical devices – Test methods of corrosive nature

[42] YY 0666 – 2008, Method forthe test of sharpness and strength of needles tips

[43] JIS T 9301: 2005, Acupuncture needle for single use

[44] 93/42/EEC, Council Directive 93/42/EEC of 14 June 1993 concerning medical devices

[45] 2007/47/EC, Directive of the European Parliament and of the Council of 5 September 2007 amending Council Directive 90/385/EEC on the approximation of the laws of the Member States relating to active implantable medical devices, Council Directive 93/42/EEC concerning medical devices and Directive 98/8/EC concerning the placing of biocidal products on the market

前　言

世界针灸学会联合会标准（以下简称"本标准"）由世界针灸学会联合会根据针灸针（特指毫针）、临床实际和医疗器械的通用要求制定。

本次修订是在世界针灸学会联合会 WFAS 标准 001：2011 基础上，根据标准化技术委员会的建议进行的，主要的变化是删除了未灭菌针灸针（专业医生在每次使用前必须消毒的多次用针灸针）的相关内容。

修订内容包括：

1. 在引言的第一段删除了未灭菌针灸针的内容。

2. 修改"1 范围"，删除未灭菌针灸针的内容。本标准适用于一次性使用无菌针灸针（特指毫针）。

3. 删除了原来条款 4.2："针灸针的品种分为未灭菌针灸针（专业医生在每次使用前必须消毒的多次用针灸针）和灭菌针灸针（一次性针灸针）两种。"

4. 修改表 5 "针体硬度"、表 7 "外观质量和表面粗糙度 Ra 值"、表 8 "穿刺力"，删除了未灭菌针灸针的内容。

5. 修改了原来条款 8.1："初包装：一次性使用无菌针灸针的无菌初包装应标示的信息。"

6. 修改了原来条款 8.2："中包装：标签内容应标示在一次性使用无菌针灸针的中包装上。"

7. 章节序号进行了调整。

本标准附录 A、附录 B 和附录 C 是规范性附录。

本标准附录 D 是资料性附录。

本标准起草单位：中国苏州医疗用品厂有限公司。

本标准主要起草人：曹炀、徐爱民、蒋心遂。

国际工作组成员：James Flowers（澳大利亚），Wu Binjiang（加拿大），Cao Yang（中国），Huang Longxiang（中国），Liu Baoyan（中国），Tan Yuansheng（中国），Denis Colin（法国），Francois Dumont（法国），Andreas Rinnoessel（德国），Sergio Bangrazi（意大利），Cho Geun Sik（韩国），Liao Chunhua（马来西亚），Liu Yun（美国）。

国际观察员：Naoto Ishizaki（日本）。

引　言

本标准涉及供专业针灸医生进行针灸疗法使用的一次性使用无菌针灸针（特指毫针）。一次性使用无菌针灸针出厂前按照已经确认过的灭菌过程进行灭菌，使产品保证无菌，专业医生可以拆开密封包装直接使用。

为避免抑制创新，本标准不限定针体直径与长度的组合。但考虑到临床的需要，标准仍要求在给出针体直径标识的同时，还要给出针体长度标识。

针灸针针尖锋利度和穿刺性能具有非常重要的临床意义，对此本标准附录 A 给出了针尖强度和锋利度指标及评价方法，本标准附录 B 给出了针尖穿刺性能定性与定量两种评价方法。

本标准附录 B 中针尖穿刺性能定性方法由于具有简单、直观、实用等特点，特别适用于过程检测和临床单位选择针灸针时的横向比较，对促进针灸针针尖质量具有非常重要的意义；针尖穿刺性能定量评价方法则为进一步评价针尖穿刺和针灸针进针性能提供方法，目前比较恰当的是采用针尖穿刺聚氨酯膜材，但该种方法目前国际上待进一步确立。考虑到未来标准的协调性，本标准以提示性的附录给出了该针尖穿刺性能评价方法，而将该条文（5.4.2）列为推荐性条文。标准中没有给出针尖穿刺聚氨酯膜材针尖锋利度指标，待将来条件成熟后再补充到标准中来。各类检验报告应包含该项性能的检验信息和结论，以利于促进产品质量的提高。

因为每个制造商的设计、生产过程和消毒灭菌方法都不同，所以未规定选用的制造针灸针针柄材料，针体和针柄材料均应具有良好的生物相容性。ISO 10993 – 1 提供了对应于医疗器械的生物学评价和试验，建议制造商在评估产品时考虑此标准的内容，以利于保证产品的安全性，促进产品质量的提高。此类评估应包括针灸针消毒灭菌工艺的影响。

同时，制造商应在产品的整个生命周期内，与国家和地区法规要求、相关的医疗器械历史数据、临床实践相结合，运用风险分析技术，对产品实施风险管理，保证产品的安全性和有效性。ISO 14971 提供了制造商对与医疗器械使用有关的风险进行有效管理的框架。

在某些国家和地区，政府法规具有法律约束力，这些要求应优先于本标准。

1 范围

本标准规定了一次性使用无菌针灸针的分类、要求、试验方法、检验规则、包装、标志、使用说明书、运输和贮存等要求。

本标准适用于供针灸疗法使用的一次性使用无菌针灸针（特指毫针）。

2 规范性引用文件

下列文件对于本文件的应用是必不可少的。凡是注日期的引用文件，其中仅注日期的版本适用于本文件。凡是不注日期的引用文件，其最新版本（包括所有的修改单）适用于本文件。

ISO/TS 15510：2007 不锈钢–化学成分

ISO 10993 – 1：2009 医疗器械生物学评价 第 1 部分：风险管理过程中的评价与试验

ISO 6507 – 1：2005 金属维氏硬度试验 第 1 部分：试验方法

ISO 11737 – 2：2007 医疗器械的消毒 微生物法 第 2 部分：灭菌验证过程的无菌检验

ISO 15223 – 1 医疗器械 用于医疗器械标签、标记和提供信息的符号 第 1 部分：通用要求

3 术语与定义

下列术语和定义适用于本标准。

3.1 针体

针灸针刺入身体的部分（图 1）。

3.2 针柄

针灸针不刺入身体的部分（图 1）。

3.3 针尖

锋利的顶端，针灸针刺入到身体的针体的末部（图 1）。

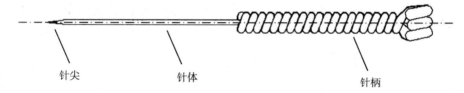

针尖　　　　　　针体　　　　　　　　　　针柄

图 1　针灸针典型结构示意图

3.4 针根

针灸针连接针体与针柄的部分（图 1）。

3.5 针尾

针柄的尾部，针尖的相反方向一端（图 1）。

3.6 无菌针灸针

已灭菌的针灸针。

3.7 未灭菌针灸针

未灭菌的针灸针。

3.8 导管

一个细长形的辅助工具，用于放置针和方便穿刺。

注：为了方便使用，针管应使用透明材料制作。

3.9 针体硬度

针灸针针体抗永久变形的特性。

3.10 初包装

第一层包裹住产品的材料。

注：初包装一般使用的是最小包装单元，直接接触一支或多支针灸针。

3.11 中包装

含一件或多件初包装的包装，用于运输和贮存。

4 分类

4.1 针灸针的典型结构和各部件名称应符合图1的规定。

4.2 针灸针的型式分为带进针管和不带进针管两种，带进针管针灸针的型式如图2所示。

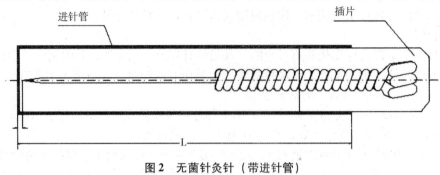

图2 无菌针灸针（带进针管）

注：图2中进针管固定方式不作统一规定。

4.3 针灸针针柄的典型型式分为环柄针、平柄针、花柄针、金属管柄针和塑料柄针等。针灸针的类型如图3所示。

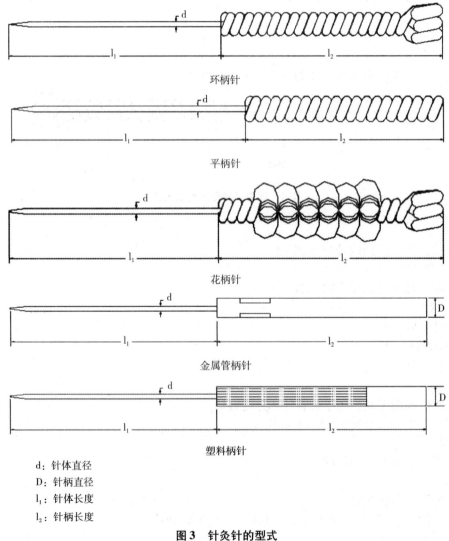

环柄针

平柄针

花柄针

金属管柄针

塑料柄针

d：针体直径
D：针柄直径
l_1：针体长度
l_2：针柄长度

图3 针灸针的型式

注：上述针型只是表明了几种特定而典型的针灸针的结构，本标准没有对套管针的固定作统一规定。

4.4 针灸针的规格以针体的直径×针体长度表示。

示例：φ0.30mm×40mm

4.5 针灸针的基本尺寸和允差应符合表1~4的规定。

4.5.1 针体直径应符合表1的规定。

表1　针体直径基本尺寸　　　　　　　（单位：mm）

标称针体直径（d）	允差
0.12≤d<0.25	±0.008
0.25≤d≤0.45	±0.015
0.45<d≤0.80	±0.020

4.5.2 针体长度应符合表2的规定。

表2　针体长度基本尺寸　　　　　　　（单位：mm）

标称针体长度（l_1）	允差
5<l_1≤25	±0.50
25<l_1≤75	±1.00
75<l_1≤100	±1.50
100<l_1≤200	±2.00

4.5.3 针灸针针柄的长度应不小于13mm。

4.5.4 绕柄金属丝应符合表3的规定；塑料柄、金属管柄等直径应符合表4的规定。

表3　绕柄金属丝直径　　　　　　　（单位：mm）

标称针体直径（d）	绕柄金属丝直径
0.12≤d<0.20	0.30
0.20≤d<0.30	0.35
0.30≤d<0.40	0.40
0.40≤d<0.50	0.45

表4　塑料柄、金属管柄等直径　　　　　　　（单位：mm）

针柄型式	针柄直径（d）
金属管柄、塑料柄等	0.80~2.50

5　要求

5.1 针灸针的基本尺寸应符合4.5条的规定。

5.2 针灸针的针体应以 ISO/TS 15510：2007 中规定的 X5CrNil8-9、X7CrNil8-9 奥氏体不锈钢制成。

注：当针灸针针体所用材料发生变化、针体表面增加涂层（如硅油润滑剂）或有迹象表明产品用于人体时发生生物安全性引起的不良反应时，应按照 ISO 10993-1：2009 的规定增加对材料和最终产品进行生物学评价，基本评价试验为：

　a. 细胞毒性；

　b. 致敏；

　c. 刺激；

　d. 环氧乙烷残留量（如采用环氧乙烷灭菌的）。

5.3 针灸针的针体硬度应符合表5的规定。

表5 针体硬度

标称针体直径（d，mm）	硬度（$HV_{0.2kg}$）
0.12≤d＜0.25	≥480，≤680
0.25≤d≤0.30	≥460，≤650
0.30＜d≤0.45	≥450，≤650
0.45＜d≤0.80	≥420，≤530

5.4 针灸针的针尖强度和穿刺性能。

5.4.1 针灸针的针尖部位应圆正不偏，无毛刺、弯钩等缺陷。应具有良好的强度，经规定的力与钢块接触顶压后，针尖不得有弯钩，其穿刺力应不大于表6的规定。

表6 顶压力和穿刺力

标称针体直径（d，mm）	顶压力（N）	穿刺力（N）
0.12≤d≤0.25	0.4	0.7
0.25＜d≤0.30	0.5	0.8
0.30＜d≤0.45	0.6	0.9
0.45＜d≤0.80	0.7	1.0

5.4.2 针灸针的针尖部位应具有良好的穿刺性能。

5.5 针体应具有良好的韧性，缠绕试验后不应有裂缝、折断和分层。

5.6 针体表面应光滑、清洁，无缺陷，无金属加工过程中的杂质。其表面外观质量和表面粗糙度参数 Ra 值应符合表7的规定。

表7 外观质量和 Ra 值

外观质量	不得有明显的伤痕、曲痕及丝纹等缺陷
Ra 值	≤0.63μm

5.7 针体与针柄的连接应牢固，在表8规定的力值下做静态拉力试验，二者的轴向位移不得大于3mm。

表8 拉力试验值

标称针体直径（d，mm）	拉力（N）
0.12≤d≤0.18	7
0.18＜d≤0.25	9
0.25＜d≤0.30	14
0.30＜d≤0.45	19
0.45＜d≤0.80	24

5.8 针灸针的针柄如采用缠绕丝，其螺旋圈应排列均匀，无明显离距。

5.9 针灸针的柄部不得有毛刺。

5.10 针灸针应平直，不得有明显的弯曲。

5.11 针灸针的柄部表面色泽应均匀。柄部如采用镀层，不得有起层、脱落现象。

5.12 针体表面如涂有润滑剂，用正常或矫正视力观察，针体外表面不应有可见的润滑剂汇聚。

5.13 针体应具有良好的耐腐蚀性能。

5.14 无菌针灸针应经一个已确认过的灭菌过程进行灭菌，使产品保证无菌。

注：适宜的灭菌方法见附录 D。ISO 11135－1：2007、ISO 11137－1：2006、ISO 17665－1：2006 规定了医疗器械灭菌过程的确认和常规控制的要求。

6 试验方法

6.1 外观

用正常或矫正视力观察，或用 10 倍放大镜检查。

6.2 表面粗糙度

用正常或矫正视力观察，或用 10 倍放大镜检查，与表面粗糙度标样进行比对。

6.3 尺寸

用通用或专用量具测量。

6.4 性能

6.4.1 硬度试验

按 ISO 6507－1：2005 的要求进行，应符合 5.3 条的规定。

6.4.2 针尖强度和锋利度、穿刺性能试验

按附录 A 的要求进行针尖强度和锋利度试验，应符合 5.4.1 条的规定。

按附录 B 的要求进行针尖穿刺性能试验，应符合 5.4.2 条的规定。

6.4.3 针体韧性试验

将针体以紧密的螺旋圈，沿螺旋线方向在一个直径为针体直径 3 倍的芯棒上缠绕，针体长度为 ≤15mm 的缠绕 2 圈，其他长度规格缠绕 5 圈，应符合 5.5 条的规定。

6.4.4 针体与针柄连接牢固度试验

先测量针体长度，然后将针体固定在夹具中，在针柄的端面上沿针体轴向缓慢施加 5.7 条规定的力，做无冲击的静态拉力试验，再测其针体长度，应符合 5.7 条的规定。

6.4.5 针柄毛刺试验

用手摸针灸针的柄部不应感觉有毛刺，应符合 5.9 条的规定。

6.4.6 针体耐腐蚀性能试验

按附录 C 的要求进行试验，应符合 5.13 条的规定。

6.4.7 无菌试验

ISO 11737－2：2007 规定了灭菌验证过程的无菌试验方法。按 ISO 11737－2：2007 的要求进行，应符合 5.14 条的规定。

7 包装

7.1 无菌针灸针的初包装应具有良好的密封性，初包装内不应有肉眼可见异物。单元包装的材料对内装物应无害，此包装的材料和设计应确保：

　　a. 在干燥、清洁和充分通风的贮存条件下，能保证内装物在使用期限内保持无菌性；

　　b. 在从包装中取出时，内装物受污染的风险最小；

　　c. 在正常的搬动、运输和贮存期间，对内装物有充分的保护；

　　d. 一旦打开，包装不能轻易地重新密封，而且应有明显的被撕开的痕迹。

注：ISO 11607 和 EN 868 系列标准提供了最终医疗器械包装材料和系统的要求，制造商在针灸针的包装设计、评估确认时应考虑此标准的内容。

7.2 初包装或单元包装应能够保证针灸针在使用期限内不生锈。

7.3 中包装是提供检验和销售的最小包装单位。

7.4 外包装应有足够的强度，充分保护产品在正常搬运、运输、储存条件下不致损坏，上面的字样或标志应能保持不因历时久而模糊不清。

8 标志、使用说明书

8.1 单支包装或单元包装的初包装

初包装上至少应有下列标志：

a. 制造厂名称和（或）商标；

b. 产品名称；

c. 规格；

d. 数量（适用于单元包装）；

e. 生产日期和（或）生产批号；

f. 灭菌方式、"无菌"等字样和（或）符号；

g. "一次性使用"字样和（或）符号；

h. 灭菌有效期限。

8.2 中包装

同型式、规格针灸针的单支包装或单元包装的初包装应装入一中包装，中包装上至少应有下列标志：

a. 制造厂名称、地址和商标；

b. 产品名称；

c. 型式、规格和数量；

d. 生产日期和（或）生产批号；

e. 按法规要求的证照号；

f. 灭菌方式、"无菌"等字样和（或）符号；

g. "一次性使用"字样和（或）符号；

h. 灭菌有效期限。

i. 若适用，针体表面用涂层（如润滑剂）的，应注明涂层名称或成分。

j. 可有警告语，如"对针灸针针体材料过敏的患者应慎用""电针可能会对针体造成腐蚀""包装破损禁止使用""用后销毁"等。

在使用前检查每一中包装完整性的警示字样，除非该警示说明已在初包装中给出。

8.3 包装上的标签、标记和提供信息的符号应符合 ISO 15223 – 1 的有关规定。

8.4 使用说明书的编写应符合法规的规定。

9 运输、贮存

9.1 运输要求按订货合同。针灸针在运输时应防止重压、高处跌落、阳光直晒和雨雪浸淋。

9.2 包装后的针灸针应贮存在相对湿度不超过80%、无腐蚀性气体和通风良好清洁的室内，并对针灸针有充分的保护。

附　录　A

（规范性附录）

针灸针针尖强度和锋利度测试

A.1　定义

针灸针针尖强度：针灸针针尖垂直作用于钢块时的抗破坏能力。

针灸针针尖锋利度：针灸针针尖垂直刺穿铝箔所需之力。

A.2　针灸针针尖强度和锋利度测定仪

仪器（图 A1）应符合下列要求，并按规定程序所批准的图样及文件制造。

A.2.1　针尖锋利度刺穿力单位以"N"表示。

A.2.2　仪器的满荷重、最小示值及速度应符合表 A1 的规定。

表 A1　仪器的满荷重、最小示值及速度

项目	标示
满荷重	1.2N
最小示值	0.01N
速度	≤0.1mm/s

A.2.3　仪器的示值误差应不大于 0.01N。

A.2.4　仪器应有校正水平和防震装置，针灸针夹具夹持针的部位应能调节，使用时应平稳。

A.2.5　仪器的传动装置应灵敏可靠，当刺穿铝箔时与电极接触，指针应自动停止。

A.2.6　仪器的起始感量应不大于 0.02N。

A.3　试验针灸针针尖强度的钢块

试验针灸针针尖强度的钢块表面应光滑，无锈蚀。

A.4　检验针灸针针尖锋利度测定仪用的铝箔

A.4.1　铝箔表面应洁净、光滑，无重叠或严重褶皱、霉斑和密集成行的砂眼。

A.4.2　铝箔为软性材料，厚度为 0.05mm，偏差为 ±0.002mm，纯度不低于 99.5%。

A.4.3　铝箔的抗拉强度不小于 $3kg/mm^2$，伸长率应不小于 3%。

A.5　试验方法

A.5.1　针尖强度试验：将试样固定于仪器上（针灸针的针尖露出固定夹具 5mm），针尖垂直作用于钢块，按 A.2.2 中规定的加力速度和加荷至本标准 5.4.1 规定的数值，保持 5～10 秒后去除负荷。然后将试样以 5 倍放大镜观察，针尖不得有弯钩；或用针尖在药棉上拖拉，不带出纤维。

A.5.2　将经过强度实验的试样针灸针夹持在针灸针夹具上，通过传动系统使针灸针逐渐加力于铝箔上，摆杆相应转动，当作用于针尖的力超过铝箔强度时，针尖即刺穿铝箔与电极接触，仪器自动停止加力。此时，摆杆上指针所指示的值即为该针尖的刺穿力。

A.5.3　按下工作控制开关按钮，使摆杆和指针复位。

A.5.4　移动铝箔夹具内的铝箔，使各刺穿孔的间距大于试样直径的 3 倍以上。

A.5.5　重复上述 A.5.2、A.5.3、A.5.4 的步骤，测定 3 次，取其算术平均值。

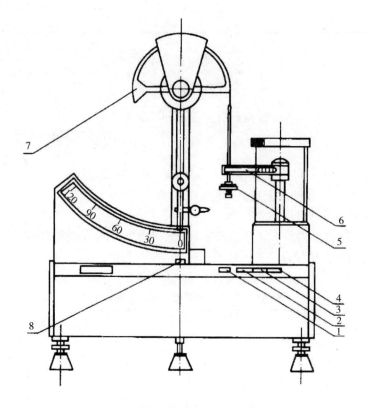

1：电源开关

2，3，4：工作控制开关

5：铝箔夹具

6：针夹

7：调节摆杆

8：水平仪

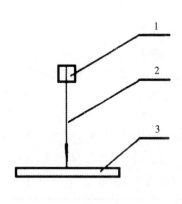 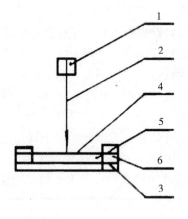

强度试验

1：夹头

2：针体

3：钢块

锋利度试验

4：穿刺材料

5：间隙

6：夹具

图 A1　针灸针针尖强度和锋利度测定仪

附 录 B

（规范性附录）

针灸针针尖穿刺性能试验方法

B.1 方法一：定性试验方法

将橡胶外科手套（符合 ISO 10282：2002）膜片蒙于一直径约 100mm 的杯口上，适当绷紧并用橡皮筋固定，持针灸针垂直对膜片进行穿刺。穿刺过程中，膜片下凹小、阻力极小、手感轻柔、声响小者，表明针尖锋利。反之，则表明针尖不锋利。

注： 此法可以凭手感对针的穿刺性能进行定性评价。适合于采购方进行横向比较以及生产过程中的质量控制。

B.2 方法二：定量试验方法

B.2.1 穿刺力评价用试验仪器

图 B1 是测量和记录穿刺力的典型仪器构成示意图，也可用具有相同性能和精度的其他装置。仪器应提供：

a. 速度 V =（50～250）mm/min，平均驱动精度 ≤ 设定驱动速度 ±5%。

b. （0～50）的传感器，平均精度为满量程的 ±5%。

c. 聚合膜夹持后穿刺直径等于 10mm。

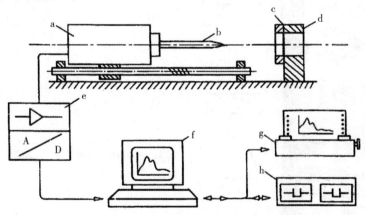

图 B1 穿刺性能评价用典型试验仪器构成示意图

B.2.2 聚合膜材料

适合于穿刺试验的聚合膜是具有弹性、厚度为 0.35 ±0.05mm、邵尔（A）硬度为 85 ±10HA 的聚氨酯膜。

B.2.3 穿刺力评价试验步骤

B.2.3.1 聚合膜在 22℃ ±2℃ 下放置 24 小时，并在相同的温度下进行试验。

B.2.3.2 将一片连续长度的聚合膜 C 的一部分竖直夹持于装置 DK，应避免聚合膜受张力。如果聚合膜具有精加工面，此面要朝向针尖。

B.2.3.3 试验用针灸针针柄装于固定装置，其针体与聚合膜的表面垂直，针尖指向供穿刺的圆形区域的中心。

B.2.3.4 移动速度设为 100mm/min。

B.2.3.5 启动试验仪器。

B.2.3.6 穿刺聚合膜，同时记录力对应于位移的曲线图。

B.2.3.7 测定相应的峰值力 F_0、F_1、F_2。

B.2.3.8 每穿刺一次聚合膜片，要选择以前没有使用和没有穿刺过的区域。

B.2.4 记录坐标图中的峰值力

针在穿刺时，可通过观察穿过聚合膜的几个典型峰值来识别各力值。

F_0：针尖刺过聚合膜时的峰值力

F_1：针尖斜面切过聚合膜时的峰值力

F_2：沿针体长度穿过聚合膜时的摩擦峰值力

B.3 结果表示

应通过与同种针（已知其质量性能）的图形比较，来评价所测得的力－位移坐标图。

B.4、B.5 给出典型坐标图，同时也给出了试验结果的报告方式。

B.4 针穿刺膜材典型特征坐标图

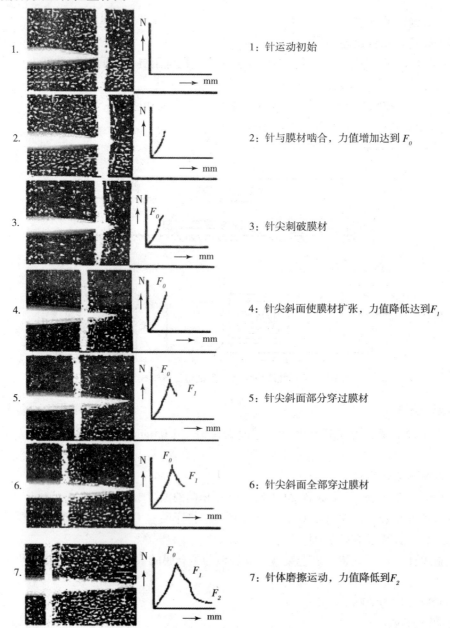

1：针运动初始

2：针与膜材啮合，力值增加达到 F_0

3：针尖刺破膜材

4：针尖斜面使膜材扩张，力值降低达到 F_1

5：针尖斜面部分穿过膜材

6：针尖斜面全部穿过膜材

7：针体磨擦运动，力值降低到 F_2

B. 5　典型的针穿刺力 F_0、F_1、F_2坐标图

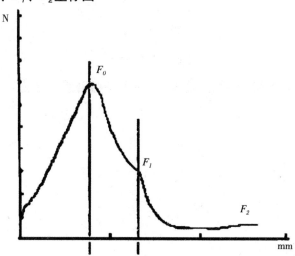

附　录　C

（规范性附录）

耐腐蚀性能试验方法——柠檬酸溶液试验法

C.1　试验器具

玻璃烧杯。

C.2　试剂

柠檬酸（化学纯）。

C.3　准备

C.3.1　试验用水

试验用水为符合 ISO 3696 规定的三级水。

C.3.2　柠檬酸溶液配制

用三级水配制 100g/L（10％）柠檬酸溶液。

C.3.3　准备

将针灸针针体或制造针体的奥氏体不锈钢材料去除油污，清洗干净，可用丙酮或其他有机溶剂浸泡或擦拭试件进行脱脂处理，用水冲洗，最后用三级水漂洗干净、备用。

C.4　试验步骤

C.4.1　将试件浸没在柠檬酸溶液中，在室温条件下保持 5 小时。

C.4.2　取出试件，用三级水冲洗。

C.4.3　试件放入盛有三级水的玻璃烧杯中煮沸 30 分钟。

C.4.4　试件在试验水中冷却，室温保持 48 小时。

C.4.5　从试验水中取出试件，置于空气中自然蒸发、干燥或用热空气吹干。

C.5　试验评价

以目力或 10 倍放大镜检查试件表面的腐蚀痕迹，其腐蚀程度应为无任何锈蚀现象。

附　录　D

（资料性附录）

文献目录

[1] ISO 780: 1997, Packaging – Pictorial marking for handling of goods

[2] ISO 2859 – 1: 1999, Sampling procedures for inspection by attributes – Part 1: Sampling schemes indexed by acceptance quality limit (AQL) for lot – by – lot inspection

[3] ISO 3696: 1987, Water for analytical laboratory use – Specification and test methods

[4] ISO 6507 – 1: 2005, Metallic materials – Vickers hardness test – Part 1: Test method

[5] ISO 6507 – 2: 2005, Metallic materials – Vickers hardness test – Part 2: Verification and calibration of testing machines

[6] ISO 6507 – 3: 2005, Metallic materials – Vickers hardness test – Part 3: Calibration of reference blocks

[7] ISO 6507 – 4: 2005, Metallic materials – Vickers hardness test – Part 4: Tables of hardness values

[8] ISO 7864: 1993, Sterile hypodermic needles for single use

[9] ISO 7000: 1989, Graphical symbols for use one equipment – Index and synopsis

[10] ISO 10282: 2002, Single – use sterile rubber surgical glovers – Specification

[11] ISO 10993 – 1: 2009, Biological evaluation of medical devices – Part 1: Evaluation and testing within a risk management process

[12] ISO 10993 – 5: 2009, Biological evaluation of medical devices – Part 5: Tests for in vitro cytotoxicity

[13] ISO 10993 – 7: 2008, Biological evaluation of medical devices – Part 7: Ethylene oxide sterilization residuals

[14] ISO 10993 – 10: 2002, Biological evaluation of medical devices – Part 10: Tests for irritation and delayed – type hypersensitivity (ISO 10993 – 10: 2002/Amd 1: 2006)

[15] ISO 10993 – 11: 2006, Biological evaluation of medical devices – Part 11: Tests for systemic toxicity

[16] ISO 11135 – 1: 2007, Sterilization of health care products – Ethylene oxide – Part 1: Requirements for development, validation and routine control of a sterilization process for medical devices

[17] ISO 11137 – 1: 2006, Sterilization of health care products – Radiation – Part 1: Requirements for development, validation and routine control of a sterilization process for medical devices

[18] ISO 11137 – 2: 2006, Sterilization of health care products – Radiation – Part 2: Establishing the sterilization dose

[19] ISO 11138 – 1: 2006, Sterilization of health care products – Biological indicators – Part 1: General requirements

[20] ISO 11138 – 2: 2006, Sterilization of health care products – Biological indicators – Part 2: Biological indicators for ethylene oxide sterilization processes

[21] ISO 11607 – 1: 2006, Packaging for terminally sterilized medical devices – Part 1: Requirements for materials, sterile barrier systems and packaging systems

[22] ISO 11607 – 2: 2006, Packaging for terminally sterilized medical devices – Part 2: Validation requirements for forming, sealing and assembly processes

[23] ISO 11737 – 1: 2006, Sterilization of medical devices – Microbiological methods – Part 1: Determination of a population of microorganisms on products

[24] ISO 11737 – 2 – 2007, Sterilization of medical devices – Microbiological methods – Part 2: Tests of sterility performed in the validation of a sterilization process

[25] ISO 13485: 2003, Medical devices – Quality management systems – Requirements for regulatory purposes

[26] ISO 14971: 2007, Medical Devices – Application of risk management to medical devices

[27] ISO 15223 – 1: 2007, Medical devices – Symbols to be used with medical device labels, labelling and information to be supplied – Part 1: General requirements

[28] ISO 15223 – 2: 2010, Medical devices – Symbols to be used with medical device labels, labelling, and information to be supplied – Part 2: Symbol development, selection and validation

[29] ISO/TS 15510: 2007, Stainless steels – Chemical composition

[30] ISO 17665 – 1: 2006, Sterilization of health care products – Moist heat – Part 1: Requirements for the development, validation and routine control of a sterilization process for medical devices

[31] EN 980: 2008, Graphical Symbols for Use in the Labelling of Medical Devices

[32] EN 1041: 2008, Information Supplied by the Manufacturer with Medical Devices

[33] EN 10088 – 1: 2005, Stainless steels

[34] GB/T 1031 – 1995, 表面粗糙度参数及其数值

[35] GB 2024 – 1994, 针灸针

[36] GB/DRT 2024 – 2010, 针灸针 (征求意见稿)

[37] GB 15811 – 2001, 一次性使用无菌注射针

[38] GB 15980 – 1995, 一次性使用医疗用品卫生标准

[39] YY 0043 – 2005, 医用缝合针

[40] YY 0033 – 2000, 无菌医疗器具生产管理规范

[41] YY/T 0149 – 2006, 不锈钢医用器械耐腐蚀性能试验方法

[42] YY 0666 – 2008, 针尖锋利度和强度试验方法

[43] JIS T 9301: 2005, Acupuncture needle for single use

[44] 93/42/EEC, Council Directive 93/42/EEC of 14 June 1993 concerning medical devices

[45] 2007/47/EC, Directive of the European Parliament and of the Council of 5 September 2007 amending Council Directive 90/385/EEC on the approximation of the laws of the Member States relating to active implantable medical devices, Council Directive 93/42/EEC concerning medical devices and Directive 98/8/EC concerning the placing of biocidal products on the market